DIABETIC RECIPES

COOKBOOK

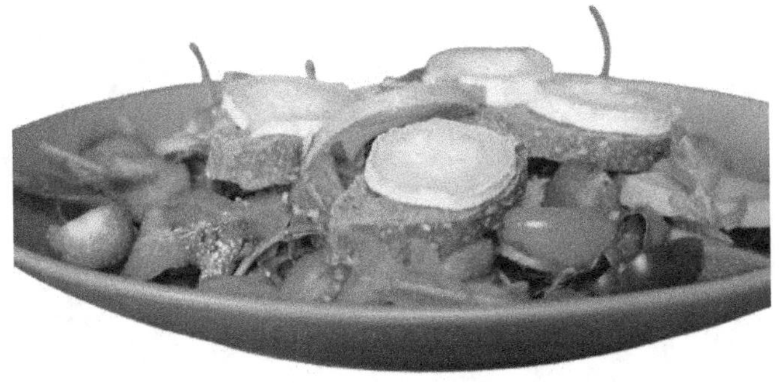

"Complete Practical Diabetic Guide on Managing Diabetes"

Valerie Hollifield

INTRODUCTION
WELCOME TO FLAVORFUL LIVING

Welcome to Flavorful Living, an enchanting journey that extends beyond the boundaries of conventional cookbooks. This collection isn't just about recipes—it's a heartfelt testament to the harmonious fusion of delectable cuisine and mindful wellness, specifically tailored for those of us navigating the intricate path of type 2 diabetes.

In my own experience, Flavorful Living has been a revelation—a culinary odyssey that rekindled my love for food while keeping my health in check. As someone who once felt that a diabetes diagnosis was a culinary sentence, this cookbook showed me that taste and nourishment can coexist in perfect harmony. The recipes not only invigorate the senses but also respect the intricate balance my body requires.

The journey begins with aromatic breakfasts that set the tone for the day ahead. From energizing smoothies that infuse life into every cell to hearty oatmeal variations that comfort the soul, each dish seems to whisper that indulgence need not compromise well-being.

However, what truly sets Flavorful Living apart is its celebration of community and shared victories. Through personal stories of individuals who have triumphed over type 2 diabetes, this cookbook is a beacon of hope. Reading about real people who've harnessed the power of flavorful, diabetes-friendly meals to transform their lives offers not only inspiration but a tangible roadmap to success.

Flavorful Living is a lifeline for those of us seeking a vibrant life without sacrificing taste. It bridges the gap between culinary artistry and the science of managing diabetes, a testimony to the fact that every meal can be a step toward both satisfaction and well-being. So, join me in savoring this journey—one that redefines what's possible at the intersection of health and flavor. Welcome to Flavorful Living, where each dish is a triumph and every bite is a celebration.

Understanding Type 2 Diabetes and Nutrition

Embarking on a journey to manage type 2 diabetes demands a deep understanding of the intricate link between your diet and your health. This chapter serves as a beacon of clarity, illuminating the path towards informed choices and better well-being.

Deciphering Type 2 Diabetes: Insights that Empower

Type 2 diabetes, a metabolic condition, hinges on how your body handles glucose—the energy sourced from food. Your ability to navigate this condition is grounded in comprehending the interplay of blood sugar levels and the nutrients you consume.

Nutrition: Beyond the Basics

Nutrition, often seen as mere sustenance, transforms into a precise science for diabetes management.

Balancing carbohydrates, proteins, fats, and fiber is pivotal, directly affecting your blood sugar levels.

Central to this understanding is the role of carbohydrates, which transform into glucose in your bloodstream. The distinction between simple and complex carbohydrates becomes vital knowledge.

Crafting Your Plate: The Plate Method

Empowering and practical, the Plate Method divides your plate into sections: half for non-starchy veggies, a quarter for lean protein, and the rest for whole grains or starchy veggies. This approach controls portions and stabilizes blood sugar by providing a balanced nutrient intake.

Glycemic Index: Navigating Carbs

The Glycemic Index (GI) rates how carbs influence blood sugar. Low-GI foods release glucose gradually, preventing spikes, while high-GI foods can trigger rapid increases. Armed with this insight, you can opt for whole grains, legumes, and fibrous veggies for sustained energy release.

Mindful Eating: A Holistic Approach

Beyond the science lies mindfulness. Savoring each bite, listening to your body, and recognizing fullness play a role. This approach cultivates a healthier relationship with food and facilitates portion control.

By grasping the intricate connection between type 2 diabetes and nutrition, you gain a powerful tool for health management. This knowledge transcends theory, guiding your practical choices. With each meal, you nurture your body, embracing a life that's not just well-informed, but also vibrant and flavorful.

Navigating Your Diabetes Journey

Your diabetes journey is uniquely yours—an opportunity to steer your health in a positive direction. Rather than a setback, consider it a catalyst for transformation. The decisions you make today shape your tomorrow, underlining your ability to influence your well-being.

Knowledge as Armor: Equipping Yourself

In this voyage, knowledge is your greatest ally. Dive into understanding diabetes intricately—its effects on your body, factors influencing blood sugar, and strategies for control. Armed with insights, you'll confidently navigate dietary choices, physical activity, medications, and lifestyle adjustments.

Strength in Numbers: Building a Support Network

Your journey isn't solitary; it's woven with threads of support. Engage your healthcare team, family, and friends. Their encouragement, wisdom, and companionship offer solace in challenges and elevate your successes.

Rising Above Challenges: Resilience in Practice

Obstacles are part of any journey, but your resilience defines your path. Elevated blood sugar readings and uncertainties are mere twists in the road. Embrace setbacks as learning opportunities, and use them to recalibrate your strategy.

Harmony of Body and Mind: Cultivating Balance

Your journey encompasses both physical and mental well-being. Implement stress-management techniques, mindfulness practices, and hobbies that kindle joy. The synergy of body and mind bolsters your journey's foundation.

Celebrating Progress: Honoring Milestones

Celebrate each achievement, regardless of size. Hitting a target blood sugar level, adopting a healthier habit, or confronting a fear signify progress. These milestones validate your commitment and propel you forward.

Your Journey's Ripple Effect: Inspiring Others

Your journey resonates beyond your experience, inspiring others to embark on their own paths to health. Your resilience and victories become a beacon of hope, showcasing the transformative power of perseverance.

Navigating your diabetes journey isn't just a passage; it's a transformative expedition enriching your life's fabric. With each stride, you sow seeds for a healthier, more vibrant future. Embrace this voyage, empower yourself with knowledge, and journey towards a life characterized by strength, well-being, and an unbreakable spirit.

CHAPTER 1: BREAKFASTS TO JUMPSTART YOUR DAY

Energizing Morning Smoothies

Ingredients: Purposeful Choices

Begin with a base—almond milk, coconut water, or Greek yogurt—for creaminess. Add:

Leafy Greens: Spinach, kale, or Swiss chard for vitamins and antioxidants.

Fruits: Berries, bananas, or mangoes for natural sweetness and vitamins.

Healthy Fats: Avocado, chia seeds, or flaxseeds for sustained energy.

Protein: Greek yogurt, tofu, or nut butter for fullness and muscle support.

Extras: Ginger, turmeric, or cinnamon for flavor and added benefits.

Nutritional Value: Nutrient Boost

Vitamins and Minerals: Leafy greens and fruits supply vital nutrients.

Fiber: Fruits and seeds aid digestion and satisfaction.

Protein: Protein sources sustain fullness and muscle strength.

Healthy Fats: Avocado and seeds provide enduring energy.

Antioxidants: Berries and vibrant ingredients guard cells.

Preparation: Streamlined Steps

Base: Choose a liquid base—water, almond milk, or coconut water.

Greens: Toss in a handful of greens for nutrition.

Fruits: Combine fruits for natural sweetness and vitamins.

Protein: Add a protein source like Greek yogurt or a plant option.

Healthy Fats: Incorporate a touch of avocado or nut butter.

Extras: Enhance with spices, seeds, or superfoods.

Blend: Blend until smooth and creamy.

Enjoy: Pour into a glass and relish your invigorating creation.

Wholesome Oatmeal Variations

Base: Nutrient-Rich Oats

Start with a foundation of oats known for their fiber, vitamins, and sustained energy release:

Old-Fashioned Rolled Oats: Classic and hearty, they provide a chewy texture.

Steel-Cut Oats: Coarse and nutty, they offer a more robust texture.

Instant Oats: Quick and convenient, they're perfect for busy mornings.

Preparation: A Blank Canvas for Creativity

Cooking Oats: Boil oats in water or milk until they reach your desired consistency.

Creamy Base: For creaminess, add mashed banana, pumpkin puree, or Greek yogurt.

Sweeteners: Opt for natural sweeteners like honey, maple syrup, or dates.

Flavor Enhancers: Infuse with vanilla extract, cinnamon, or a pinch of nutmeg.

Top with Texture: Add crunch with nuts, seeds, or granola.

Fruits: Fresh berries, sliced banana, diced apple, or dried fruits add natural sweetness and vitamins.

Protein Boost: Stir in nut butter, chia seeds, or a sprinkle of protein powder.

Nutritional Benefits: Balancing Flavor and Health

Fiber: Oats contribute soluble fiber, aiding digestion and promoting fullness.

Complex Carbs: Oats provide sustained energy due to their complex carbohydrate content.

Vitamins and Minerals: Fresh fruits and add-ons offer an array of vitamins and minerals.

Protein: Enhancements like nut butter and seeds elevate protein content.

Versatility: Tailored to You

Create oatmeal that suits your taste preferences and dietary needs:

Classic: Enjoy plain oats with a touch of honey and fruits for a simple start.

Nutty Delight: Add almond butter, chopped nuts, and sliced bananas for a nutty twist.

Berry Bliss: Mix in fresh berries and a drizzle of maple syrup for fruity goodness.

Pumpkin Spice: Embrace the season with pumpkin puree, cinnamon, and a sprinkle of nutmeg.

Overnight Oats: Prepare the night before with milk, yogurt, and toppings for a grab-and-go option.

Hearty Vegetable Frittata

Ingredients: A Symphony of Flavors

Gather an array of fresh ingredients for your frittata:

Eggs: The heart of the frittata, providing protein and a rich texture.

Vegetables: Choose an assortment of bell peppers, spinach, onions, and zucchini for color, vitamins, and fiber.

Cheese: Opt for low-fat cheese like feta or cheddar to enhance flavor and creaminess.

Herbs and Spices: Fresh herbs like parsley or thyme, along with spices like black pepper and a pinch of nutmeg, add depth and aroma.

Milk: A splash of milk contributes to the fluffiness of the frittata.

Preparation: Crafting Your Culinary Canvas

Sauté Vegetables: In an oven-safe skillet, sauté the vegetables until tender and slightly caramelized.

Whisk Eggs: In a bowl, whisk eggs, milk, and a pinch of salt until well combined.

Combine Ingredients: Pour the egg mixture over the sautéed vegetables in the skillet.

Add Cheese and Herbs: Sprinkle cheese and fresh herbs evenly over the mixture.

Cook on Stovetop: Cook on low heat until the edges are set but the center is still slightly liquid.

Bake: Transfer the skillet to a preheated oven and bake until the frittata is fully set and golden on top.

Serve and Enjoy: Carefully remove from the oven, slice into wedges, and serve warm.

Nutritional Benefits: Balancing Flavor and Health

Protein: Eggs provide high-quality protein for satiety and muscle health.

Vegetables: Colorful vegetables contribute vitamins, minerals, and antioxidants.

Fiber: Vegetables supply dietary fiber, aiding digestion and promoting fullness.

Low Carbs: This dish is relatively low in carbohydrates, making it suitable for balanced meals.

Fluffy Whole Wheat Pancakes

Ingredients: The Essentials for Wholesome Goodness

Whole Wheat Flour: Rich in fiber and nutrients, whole wheat flour forms the heart of these pancakes.

Baking Powder: Provides the fluffiness that makes these pancakes irresistible.

Salt: Enhances flavor and balances the sweetness.

Milk: Choose your preferred milk—dairy or plant-based—for the perfect consistency.

Egg: Adds structure and protein to the pancakes.

Sweetener: Opt for honey, maple syrup, or a healthier sweetener of your choice.

Oil: A touch of oil keeps the pancakes moist and prevents sticking.

Preparation: Crafting Fluffy Pancake Perfection

Mix Dry Ingredients: In a bowl, combine whole wheat flour, baking powder, and a pinch of salt.

Whisk Wet Ingredients: In a separate bowl, whisk together milk, egg, sweetener, and oil.

Combine: Gently fold the wet ingredients into the dry mixture until just combined. Don't overmix; a few lumps are okay.

Rest the Batter: Let the batter rest for a few minutes to allow the baking powder to activate.

Cooking: Heat a skillet over medium heat and lightly grease with oil or cooking spray. Pour 1/4 cup of batter for each pancake.

Flip and Cook: When bubbles form on the surface, flip the pancake and cook until golden on both sides.

Serve and Enjoy: Stack your fluffy whole wheat pancakes, top with fresh fruits, a drizzle of honey, or a dollop of Greek yogurt.

Nutritional Benefits: Balancing Flavor and Nutrients

Fluffy whole wheat pancakes offer a fusion of taste and health:

Whole Grains: Whole wheat flour provides fiber and essential nutrients.

Protein: Eggs and milk contribute protein, aiding in muscle health and satiety.

Fiber: Whole grains supply dietary fiber for digestion and fullness.

Moderate Sweetness: Using natural sweeteners keeps sugar content in check.

Versatility: Personalize Your Pancakes

Experiment with variations to suit your preferences:

Add-Ins: Incorporate blueberries, mashed banana, or chopped nuts into the batter.

Spices: Sprinkle cinnamon or nutmeg for an aromatic twist.

Toppings: Top with fresh berries, sliced banana, or a dusting of powdered sugar.

Creamy Tomato Basil Soup

Ingredients: The Essence of Flavor

Tomatoes: Opt for canned or fresh tomatoes for a rich tomato base.

Onion and Garlic: These aromatic additions infuse depth and warmth.

Fresh Basil: Fragrant basil leaves provide an irresistible herbaceous note.

Vegetable Broth: The foundation of the soup's savory essence.

Heavy Cream: For velvety creaminess and luscious texture.

Butter: A touch of butter enriches the soup's flavor.

Seasonings: Salt, black pepper, and a pinch of red pepper flakes for a hint of heat.

Preparation: Crafting Culinary Excellence

Sauté Aromatics: In a pot, sauté chopped onion and minced garlic in butter until fragrant and translucent.

Add Tomatoes: Pour in the tomatoes and cook until softened, breaking them down with a spoon.

Simmer: Add vegetable broth and bring to a gentle simmer. Let the flavors meld.

Blend: Use an immersion blender to purée the soup until smooth. Alternatively, transfer to a regular blender in batches.

Creamy Indulgence: Pour in heavy cream, stirring to achieve the desired creamy consistency.

Basil Infusion: Stir in fresh basil leaves for a burst of aromatic freshness.

Season and Serve: Season with salt, black pepper, and red pepper flakes. Ladle into bowls and garnish with additional basil.

Nutritional Benefits: Balancing Indulgence and Health

Creamy tomato basil soup offers a fusion of satisfaction and nutrition:

Tomatoes: Rich in antioxidants like lycopene, tomatoes contribute to heart health.

Fresh Basil: Basil brings vitamins and adds a refreshing aroma.

Cream and Butter: While adding indulgence, these ingredients provide richness to savor in moderation.

Vegetable Broth: A foundation of flavors without unnecessary added fats.

Versatility: Pair and Enjoy

Pair your soup with crusty bread, a side salad, or even a grilled cheese sandwich for a complete meal.

Mediterranean Chickpea Salad

Ingredients: A Tapestry of Freshness

Chickpeas: A hearty base rich in protein and fiber.

Colorful Vegetables: Choose a medley of cucumbers, cherry tomatoes, red onion, and bell peppers for vibrancy and nutrients.

Kalamata Olives: For a burst of briny flavor and healthy fats.

Feta Cheese: Provides a creamy and tangy element.

Fresh Herbs: Include parsley and mint for an aromatic flourish.

Lemon: A zesty citrus kick that brightens the salad.

Extra Virgin Olive Oil: Drizzle for richness and the characteristic Mediterranean touch.

Seasonings: Salt, black pepper, and a dash of dried oregano for depth.

Preparation: Crafting Mediterranean Magic

Prepare Chickpeas: Rinse and drain canned chickpeas or cook dried chickpeas until tender.

Chop Vegetables: Dice cucumbers, halve cherry tomatoes, finely slice red onion, and dice bell peppers.

Assemble: In a bowl, combine chickpeas, vegetables, and Kalamata olives.

Add Cheese and Herbs: Crumble feta cheese over the mixture and sprinkle with chopped parsley and mint.

Zest and Juice: Zest and juice a lemon over the salad for a refreshing tang.

Drizzle Olive Oil: Gently drizzle extra virgin olive oil for richness and Mediterranean flavor.

Season and Toss: Sprinkle with salt, black pepper, and dried oregano. Gently toss to combine.

Chill and Serve: Refrigerate the salad for an hour to let the flavors meld. Serve as a main or side dish.

Nutritional Benefits: A Bounty of Goodness

Mediterranean chickpea salad offers a tapestry of nutrition:

Chickpeas: Protein, fiber, and essential minerals.

Vegetables: A rainbow of vitamins, minerals, and antioxidants.

Feta Cheese: Calcium and a touch of healthy fats.

Olive Oil: Monounsaturated fats and antioxidants.

Fresh Herbs: Aromatic compounds and additional vitamins.

Versatility: A Complete Meal or Side Dish

Enjoy your Mediterranean chickpea salad as a hearty main dish or a refreshing side alongside grilled meats or fish.

Roasted Vegetable Quinoa Salad

Ingredients: A Symphony of Nutrients

Quinoa: A protein-packed ancient grain with a delicate texture.

Assorted Vegetables: Choose a medley of bell peppers, zucchini, cherry tomatoes, and red onion for variety and color.

Olive Oil: For roasting vegetables to perfection and adding richness.

Fresh Herbs: Opt for parsley, basil, or cilantro for a burst of freshness.

Lemon: A zesty citrus note that brightens the dish.

Crumbled Feta Cheese: Provides a creamy and tangy element.

Nuts or Seeds: Toasted pine nuts, almonds, or sunflower seeds for added crunch.

Seasonings: Salt, black pepper, and a touch of dried oregano for depth.

Preparation: Crafting Culinary Excellence

Cook Quinoa: Rinse quinoa and cook according to package instructions until fluffy and tender.

Roast Vegetables: Toss chopped vegetables with olive oil, salt, and pepper. Roast until caramelized and slightly crispy.

Chop Herbs: Finely chop fresh herbs for an aromatic touch.

Assemble: In a large bowl, combine cooked quinoa, roasted vegetables, and crumbled feta cheese.

Zest and Juice: Zest the lemon over the mixture and drizzle with its juice.

Add Crunch: Sprinkle toasted nuts or seeds for delightful texture.

Season and Toss: Season with salt, black pepper, and dried oregano. Gently toss to combine.

Serve and Enjoy: Portion the salad into bowls and relish the vibrant flavors.

Nutritional Benefits: Balance and Wholesomeness

Roasted vegetable quinoa salad offers a balanced spectrum of nutrients:

Quinoa: Plant-based protein, dietary fiber, and essential amino acids.

Vegetables: Vitamins, minerals, and antioxidants from a variety of colorful vegetables.

Olive Oil: Healthy monounsaturated fats and antioxidant compounds.

Feta Cheese: Creaminess, protein, and a touch of tang.

Nuts or Seeds: Additional protein, healthy fats, and crunch.

Versatility: A Meal or Side Dish

Enjoy your roasted vegetable quinoa salad as a satisfying main dish or a side alongside grilled proteins.

Spicy Lentil and Spinach Soup

Ingredients: A Fusion of Flavors

Gather the essentials for a flavorful and satisfying experience:

Lentils: Opt for brown or green lentils for their earthy taste and hearty texture.

Fresh Spinach: Packed with vitamins and minerals, spinach adds vibrancy.

Onion and Garlic: Aromatic essentials that infuse depth and warmth.

Tomatoes: Canned or fresh tomatoes provide a rich base for the soup.

Vegetable Broth: The foundation of the soup's savory essence.

Spices: Red pepper flakes, cumin, and paprika for a spicy kick and complexity.

Lemon: A zesty touch that balances the flavors.

Olive Oil: For sautéing and richness.

Seasonings: Salt, black pepper, and a dash of turmeric for depth.

Preparation: Crafting Culinary Warmth

Sauté Aromatics: In a pot, sauté chopped onion and minced garlic in olive oil until fragrant.

Spice it Up: Add cumin, paprika, and red pepper flakes. Sauté for another minute.

Add Lentils and Tomatoes: Stir in lentils and tomatoes. Cook for a few minutes to infuse flavors.

Simmer: Pour in vegetable broth and bring to a gentle simmer. Allow lentils to cook until tender.

Add Spinach: Add fresh spinach and cook until wilted.

Lemon Zest and Juice: Zest the lemon over the soup and drizzle with its juice.

Season and Serve: Season with salt, black pepper, and a pinch of turmeric for color. Ladle into bowls and savor the warmth.

Nutritional Benefits: A Hearty Blend

Spicy lentil and spinach soup offers a blend of robust flavors and nutrition:

Lentils: Protein, dietary fiber, and essential minerals.

Spinach: Vitamins A and K, iron, and antioxidants.

Tomatoes: Vitamins, lycopene, and a natural umami base.

Spices: Antioxidants and potential health benefits from spices like cumin.

Olive Oil: Healthy monounsaturated fats and richness.

Versatility: A Satisfying Meal

Enjoy your spicy lentil and spinach soup as a wholesome and filling meal. Pair with crusty bread for a complete experience.

CHAPTER 3: WHOLESOME MAIN DISHES

Baked Herb-Crusted Salmon

Ingredients: An Array of Flavors

Salmon Fillets: Choose fresh salmon fillets for their tender texture and rich flavor.

Fresh Herbs: Opt for a combination of parsley, dill, thyme, or rosemary for a burst of herbal aromas.

Breadcrumbs: Fine breadcrumbs provide a delicate crunch and help hold the herb crust.

Lemon Zest: For a zesty brightness that complements the richness of the salmon.

Garlic: Minced garlic adds depth and complexity to the crust.

Dijon Mustard: Provides a tangy kick and helps bind the herb mixture.

Olive Oil: Drizzling of olive oil adds moisture and richness.

Salt and Pepper: For balanced seasoning.

Preparation: Crafting Culinary Elegance

Prepare Herb Mixture: In a bowl, combine finely chopped fresh herbs, breadcrumbs, lemon zest, minced garlic, Dijon mustard, and a drizzle of olive oil. Mix until the mixture resembles coarse crumbs.

Season Salmon: Pat the salmon fillets dry and season with salt and pepper on both sides.

Coat with Herb Crust: Press the herb mixture onto the top surface of each salmon fillet, creating a generous crust.

Baking: Place the herb-crusted salmon fillets on a baking sheet lined with parchment paper. Bake in a preheated oven at 400°F (200°C) for about 12-15 minutes, or until the salmon is cooked through and flakes easily with a fork.

Serve and Enjoy: Carefully transfer the herb-crusted salmon to plates and serve hot.

Nutritional Benefits: Balance and Richness

Baked herb-crusted salmon offers a balance of flavors and nutrients:

Salmon: A rich source of omega-3 fatty acids and high-quality protein.

Fresh Herbs: Vitamins, minerals, and antioxidants from a variety of herbs.

Lemon Zest: Zesty brightness and vitamin C.

Olive Oil: Healthy monounsaturated fats and richness.

Versatility: A Culinary Delight

Enjoy your baked herb-crusted salmon as the star of a fine dining experience. Serve with roasted vegetables, steamed asparagus, or a quinoa salad for a complete meal.

Zucchini Noodles with Pesto and Cherry Tomatoes

Ingredients: A Symphony of Tastes

Zucchini: Spiralized zucchini creates tender and refreshing "noodles."

Pesto: Opt for homemade or store-bought pesto for its vibrant herbaceousness.

Cherry Tomatoes: These little gems add a burst of sweet juiciness.

Fresh Basil: For an additional layer of aromatic freshness.

Parmesan Cheese: Grated Parmesan brings a nutty and savory note.

Pine Nuts: Toasted pine nuts contribute a delightful crunch.

Lemon Zest: Adds a zesty and bright kick.

Olive Oil: Drizzle for richness and depth.

Salt and Black Pepper: To balance and enhance flavors.

Preparation: Crafting Culinary Zest

Prepare Zucchini Noodles: Spiralize the zucchini into "noodles" and set aside.

Chop Cherry Tomatoes: Halve or quarter the cherry tomatoes for easy bites.

Toss with Pesto: In a large bowl, gently toss the zucchini noodles with the pesto until well coated.

Add Tomatoes and Basil: Add the chopped cherry tomatoes and torn basil leaves to the bowl. Gently mix to combine.

Serve and Garnish: Portion the zucchini noodle mixture onto plates. Sprinkle with grated Parmesan, toasted pine nuts, and a drizzle of olive oil.

Zest and Enjoy: Zest lemon over the dish for a zesty touch. Serve as a light and refreshing meal.

Nutritional Benefits: Lightness and Flavor

Zucchini noodles with pesto and cherry tomatoes offer a harmonious blend of nutrition and taste:

Zucchini: A low-carb alternative to pasta, rich in vitamins and minerals.

Pesto: Healthy fats, vitamins, and aromatic herbs.

Cherry Tomatoes: Vitamins, antioxidants, and natural sweetness.

Basil and Lemon Zest: Freshness and zestiness that elevate the dish.

Versatility: A Refreshing Bite

Enjoy your zucchini noodles with pesto and cherry tomatoes as a light lunch or a refreshing dinner option. It's also a fantastic side dish for grilled proteins.

Grilled Chicken with Citrus Glaze

Ingredients: A Fusion of Flavors

Chicken Breasts: Choose boneless, skinless chicken breasts for a lean and tender result.

Citrus Fruits: Opt for a combination of oranges, lemons, and limes for a medley of flavors.

Honey: For a touch of natural sweetness in the glaze.

Garlic: Minced garlic adds depth and complexity.

Fresh Herbs: Choose rosemary or thyme for an aromatic flourish.

Olive Oil: Drizzle for moisture and richness.

Salt and Black Pepper: To enhance and balance flavors.

Preparation: Crafting Culinary Zest

Prepare Citrus Glaze: In a bowl, combine the juice of citrus fruits, honey, minced garlic, chopped herbs, olive oil, salt, and black pepper. Mix well to create the glaze.

Marinate Chicken: Place the chicken breasts in a sealable plastic bag or a shallow dish. Pour the citrus glaze over the chicken, ensuring it's well coated. Seal the bag or cover the dish and marinate in the refrigerator for at least 30 minutes, or ideally a few hours.

Grill: Preheat the grill to medium-high heat. Remove the chicken from the marinade, allowing any excess to drip off.

Grill Chicken: Grill the chicken breasts for about 6-7 minutes per side, or until the internal temperature reaches 165°F (74°C) and the chicken is cooked through with no pinkness.

Brush with Glaze: During the last few minutes of grilling, brush the chicken with some of the reserved citrus glaze, allowing it to caramelize and infuse the chicken with flavor.

Serve and Enjoy: Transfer the grilled chicken with citrus glaze to plates and garnish with additional chopped herbs. Serve alongside your favorite sides.

Nutritional Benefits: Flavorful Fusion

Grilled chicken with citrus glaze offers a fusion of succulence and tang:

Chicken Breasts: Lean protein that's rich in essential amino acids.

Citrus Fruits: Vitamins, antioxidants, and a burst of refreshing flavor.

Honey: A natural sweetener that balances the tanginess of the citrus.

Fresh Herbs and Olive Oil: Aromatic and healthy fats that enhance the dish.

Versatility: A Culinary Adventure

Enjoy your grilled chicken with citrus glaze as the centerpiece of a delicious meal. Serve with grilled vegetables, a refreshing salad, or a side of quinoa for a complete dining experience.

Black Bean and Sweet Potato Enchiladas

Ingredients: A Medley of Delights

Black Beans: Opt for cooked or canned black beans for their creamy texture and protein-packed goodness.

Sweet Potatoes: Roasted or boiled sweet potatoes provide natural sweetness and depth.

Tortillas: Choose corn or whole wheat tortillas for a wholesome base.

Enchilada Sauce: Either store-bought or homemade, red or green, for saucy richness.

Cheese: Shredded Monterey Jack or cheddar cheese for melty goodness.

Onion and Garlic: Minced onion and garlic for savory depth.

Spices: Ground cumin, chili powder, and paprika for a kick of flavor.

Fresh Cilantro: Chopped cilantro for an aromatic flourish.

Olive Oil: For sautéing and richness.

Salt and Black Pepper: To enhance and balance flavors.

Preparation: Crafting Culinary Fiesta

Prepare Filling: In a pan, sauté minced onion and garlic in olive oil until fragrant. Add cooked black beans and diced sweet potatoes. Sprinkle with ground cumin, chili powder, paprika, salt, and black pepper. Sauté until flavors meld and sweet potatoes are tender.

Assemble Enchiladas: Lay out tortillas and divide the black bean and sweet potato mixture among them.

Roll the tortillas and place them seam-side down in a baking dish.

Pour Enchilada Sauce: Pour the enchilada sauce over the rolled tortillas, covering them generously.

Add Cheese: Sprinkle shredded cheese over the enchiladas for a delightful melt.

Bake: Place the baking dish in a preheated oven at 350°F (175°C) for about 20-25 minutes, or until the cheese is bubbly and golden.

Garnish and Serve: Remove from the oven and garnish with chopped cilantro. Serve the enchiladas hot.

Nutritional Benefits: Hearty and Wholesome

Black bean and sweet potato enchiladas offer a harmonious blend of nutrition and taste:

Black Beans: Protein, fiber, and essential nutrients.

Sweet Potatoes: Vitamins A and C, fiber, and natural sweetness.

Tortillas: Carbohydrates and a wholesome base.

Enchilada Sauce and Cheese: Flavorful richness and indulgence.

Versatility: A Festive Meal

Enjoy your black bean and sweet potato enchiladas as a festive and satisfying meal. Serve with a side of Mexican rice, guacamole, and a fresh salad for a complete fiesta experience.

CHAPTER 4: FLAVORFUL SIDE DISHES

Lemon Garlic Roasted Brussels Sprouts

Ingredients: A Fusion of Freshness

Gather the essentials for a symphony of flavors:

Brussels Sprouts: Choose fresh Brussels sprouts, trimmed and halved, for a tender and crisp result.

Lemon: Zest and juice of lemon for a zesty kick and bright aroma.

Garlic: Minced garlic adds depth and complexity.

Olive Oil: Drizzle for roasting and richness.

Salt and Black Pepper: To enhance and balance flavors.

Red Pepper Flakes: For a hint of heat (optional).

Parmesan Cheese: Grated Parmesan adds a nutty and savory touch.

Fresh Parsley: Chopped parsley for an aromatic flourish.

Preparation: Crafting Culinary Excellence

Toss with Marinade: In a bowl, combine halved Brussels sprouts with minced garlic, olive oil, salt, black pepper, and optional red pepper flakes. Toss to coat the sprouts evenly with the marinade.

Roast: Spread the Brussels sprouts on a baking sheet in a single layer. Roast in a preheated oven at 400°F (200°C) for about 20-25 minutes, or until they are tender and have a crisp exterior.

Zest and Drizzle: Once the Brussels sprouts are roasted, zest the lemon over them and drizzle with its juice for a burst of citrus flavor.

Add Cheese: Sprinkle the roasted Brussels sprouts with grated Parmesan cheese for a delightful melt.

Garnish and Serve: Remove from the oven and garnish with chopped fresh parsley. Serve the lemon garlic roasted Brussels sprouts hot.

Nutritional Benefits: Brightness and Balance

Lemon garlic roasted Brussels sprouts offer a fusion of flavors and nutrition:

Brussels Sprouts: Vitamins C and K, fiber, and antioxidants.

Lemon: Vitamin C, zesty freshness, and brightness.

Garlic: Flavor depth and potential health benefits.

Olive Oil: Healthy monounsaturated fats and richness.

Versatility: A Culinary Delight

Enjoy your lemon garlic roasted Brussels sprouts as a side dish that complements a variety of meals. Pair them with grilled proteins, roasted chicken, or even pasta for a burst of flavor.

Quinoa and Vegetable Stir-Fry

Ingredients: A Medley of Goodness

Quinoa: Cooked quinoa serves as the hearty base, providing protein and fiber.

Assorted Vegetables: Choose a mix of bell peppers, broccoli florets, carrots, snap peas, and any other favorites for vibrant colors and textures.

Soy Sauce: For savory umami and a touch of saltiness.

Garlic and Ginger: Minced garlic and grated ginger add depth and warmth.

Sesame Oil: A drizzle of sesame oil contributes nutty richness.

Sesame Seeds: Toasted sesame seeds for a delightful crunch.

Green Onions: Sliced green onions for a fresh bite.

Red Pepper Flakes: Optional for a hint of heat.

Lime: Lime juice for a zesty kick.

Salt and Black Pepper: To enhance and balance flavors.

Preparation: Crafting Culinary Balance

Sauté Aromatics: In a pan or wok, heat a splash of sesame oil over medium heat. Add minced garlic and grated ginger. Sauté for a minute until fragrant.

Add Vegetables: Toss in the assorted vegetables, starting with those that take longer to cook (e.g., carrots, broccoli). Stir-fry until they start to soften but still have a vibrant crunch.

Stir in Quinoa: Add the cooked quinoa to the pan. Stir-fry to combine and heat through.

Season and Sauce: Drizzle soy sauce over the stir-fry for flavor. Add a pinch of red pepper flakes if desired. Season with black pepper and a touch of salt.

Finish and Zest: Squeeze lime juice over the stir-fry and toss to incorporate. Sprinkle toasted sesame seeds over the mixture.

Serve and Garnish: Transfer the quinoa and vegetable stir-fry to plates. Garnish with sliced green onions for a fresh touch.

Nutritional Benefits: Nutrient-Rich Delight

Quinoa and vegetable stir-fry offers a combination of health and flavor:

Quinoa: Protein, fiber, essential amino acids, and nutrients.

Assorted Vegetables: Vitamins, minerals, antioxidants, and vibrant colors.

Soy Sauce and Sesame Oil: Umami richness and depth of flavor.

Versatility: A Balanced Meal

Enjoy your quinoa and vegetable stir-fry as a balanced and satisfying meal on its own. Alternatively, serve it as a side dish alongside grilled proteins or tofu.

Garlic and Herb Cauliflower Mash

Ingredients: A Fusion of Flavors

Cauliflower: Choose fresh cauliflower florets for their mild taste and creamy texture when cooked.

Garlic: Minced garlic adds depth and complexity.

Fresh Herbs: Opt for a blend of chopped fresh herbs such as parsley, chives, or thyme for an aromatic flourish.

Butter: For richness and flavor.

Milk: Choose your preferred milk (dairy or plant-based) for creaminess.

Parmesan Cheese: Grated Parmesan brings a nutty and savory note.

Olive Oil: Drizzle for added richness and depth.

Salt and Black Pepper: To enhance and balance flavors.

Preparation: Crafting Culinary Comfort

Steam Cauliflower: Steam the cauliflower florets until they are tender and can be easily pierced with a fork. Drain any excess moisture.

Sauté Garlic: In a pan, sauté minced garlic in a bit of butter or olive oil until fragrant.

Blend and Mash: In a food processor or using a potato masher, combine the steamed cauliflower, sautéed garlic, chopped herbs, butter, milk, grated Parmesan, salt, and black pepper. Blend or mash until smooth and creamy. Adjust the consistency by adding more milk if needed.

Taste and Adjust: Taste the cauliflower mash and adjust the seasonings to your preference. Add more salt, pepper, or herbs as desired.

Serve and Enjoy: Transfer the garlic and herb cauliflower mash to a serving bowl. Garnish with additional chopped herbs and a drizzle of olive oil. Serve hot.

Nutritional Benefits: Creamy and Nutritious

Garlic and herb cauliflower mash offers a blend of creaminess and nutrition:

Cauliflower: Low in calories and carbs, high in vitamins C and K, and a good source of fiber.

Garlic and Herbs: Flavor depth and potential health benefits.

Butter and Milk: Creaminess and richness.

Parmesan Cheese: A nutty and savory touch.

Versatility: A Comforting Side

Enjoy your garlic and herb cauliflower mash as a comforting and nutritious side dish. Serve it alongside roasted proteins, grilled vegetables, or your favorite main course.

Brown Rice Pilaf with Mixed Herbs

Ingredients: A Medley of Aromas

Brown Rice: Choose whole grain brown rice for its nutty taste and chewy texture.

Mixed Herbs: Opt for a combination of fresh herbs such as parsley, thyme, rosemary, and chives for an aromatic flourish.

Onion: Finely chopped onion adds sweetness and depth.

Garlic: Minced garlic contributes depth and complexity.

Vegetable Broth: For a flavorful base that infuses the rice.

Olive Oil: Drizzle for richness and depth.

Salt and Black Pepper: To enhance and balance flavors.

Preparation: Crafting Herbal Delight

Sauté Aromatics: In a pot, heat a drizzle of olive oil over medium heat. Add the finely chopped onion and sauté until translucent.

Toast Rice: Add the brown rice to the pot and sauté for a couple of minutes, allowing it to slightly toast.

Add Garlic: Stir in the minced garlic and sauté for another minute until fragrant.

Simmer: Pour in the vegetable broth and bring the mixture to a gentle simmer. Cover the pot and let the rice cook until tender and the liquid is absorbed.

Fluff and Herb Infusion: Once the rice is cooked, fluff it with a fork. Gently fold in the chopped mixed herbs to infuse the rice with their aromatic flavors.

Season and Serve: Season the brown rice pilaf with salt and black pepper to taste. Transfer to a serving dish and enjoy.

Nutritional Benefits: Wholesome and Aromatic

Brown rice pilaf with mixed herbs offers a balance of wholesomeness and herbal goodness:

Brown Rice: Whole grains, fiber, and essential nutrients.

Mixed Herbs: Vitamins, minerals, antioxidants, and aromatic infusion.

Onion and Garlic: Flavor depth and potential health benefits.

Vegetable Broth: Flavorful and nutrient-rich base.

Versatility: A Flavorful Accompaniment

Enjoy your brown rice pilaf with mixed herbs as a flavorful and aromatic side dish. Serve it alongside grilled proteins, roasted vegetables, or your favorite main course.

Cucumber and Greek Yogurt Dip

Ingredients: A Fusion of Freshness

Cucumber: Choose a fresh cucumber, peeled and finely diced, for a refreshing crunch.

Greek Yogurt: Opt for thick and creamy Greek yogurt for a tangy and luxurious base.

Fresh Herbs: Select dill or mint for an aromatic flourish that complements the cucumber.

Garlic: Minced garlic adds depth and subtle pungency.

Lemon: Zest and juice of lemon for a zesty brightness.

Extra Virgin Olive Oil: Drizzle for richness and depth.

Salt and Black Pepper: To enhance and balance flavors.

Preparation: Crafting Culinary Refreshment

Prepare Cucumber: Finely dice the peeled cucumber. Place the diced cucumber in a strainer and sprinkle a pinch of salt over it. Allow it to drain for about 10 minutes to remove excess moisture.

Combine Ingredients: In a mixing bowl, combine the drained diced cucumber, Greek yogurt, minced garlic, chopped fresh herbs, lemon zest, and a squeeze of lemon juice. Mix well to combine.

Season and Chill: Season the cucumber and Greek yogurt dip with salt and black pepper to taste. Drizzle with a bit of extra virgin olive oil for added richness. Cover the bowl and refrigerate the dip for at least 30 minutes to let the flavors meld.

Serve and Enjoy: Transfer the chilled cucumber and Greek yogurt dip to a serving bowl. Garnish with additional chopped herbs and a drizzle of olive oil. Serve the dip with an array of fresh vegetables, pita bread, or as a condiment for grilled meats.

Nutritional Benefits: Cooling and Creamy

Cucumber and Greek yogurt dip offers a blend of refreshment and nutrition:

Cucumber: Hydration, vitamins, minerals, and a refreshing crunch.

Greek Yogurt: Protein, probiotics, and tangy creaminess.

Fresh Herbs and Lemon: Aromatic freshness and zesty brightness.

Versatility: A Versatile Dip

Enjoy your cucumber and Greek yogurt dip as a refreshing and versatile appetizer. It's also a great addition to picnics, parties, or as a healthy snack.

Spiced Roasted Nuts

Ingredients: A Symphony of Spices

Mixed Nuts: Choose a variety of raw nuts such as almonds, walnuts, pecans, and cashews for a rich and diverse crunch.

Spice Blend: Opt for a mix of warm spices like cumin, paprika, cayenne pepper, and a touch of cinnamon for a balanced kick.

Honey or Maple Syrup: For a touch of natural sweetness and to help the spices adhere.

Olive Oil: Drizzle for roasting and a hint of richness.

Salt: To enhance and balance flavors.

Fresh Herbs: Optional chopped fresh herbs like rosemary or thyme for an aromatic touch.

Preparation: Crafting Culinary Temptation

Prepare Spice Blend: In a bowl, mix the spice blend, combining cumin, paprika, a pinch of cayenne pepper, and a hint of cinnamon. Adjust the spice levels to your preference.

Coat Nuts: In a separate bowl, toss the mixed nuts with a drizzle of olive oil to coat them lightly. Add the spice blend and toss again to evenly coat the nuts with the aromatic spices.

Sweet and Salty Balance: Drizzle honey or maple syrup over the spiced nuts, stirring gently to ensure they are lightly sweetened. Sprinkle with a bit of salt to balance the flavors.

Roast: Spread the coated nuts in a single layer on a baking sheet lined with parchment paper. Roast in a preheated oven at 350°F (175°C) for about 10-15 minutes, or until the nuts are golden and fragrant.

Cool and Crisp: Once roasted, allow the spiced nuts to cool completely on the baking sheet. This will help them crisp up even further as they cool.

Garnish and Serve: Transfer the spiced roasted nuts to a serving bowl. If desired, sprinkle with chopped fresh herbs for an aromatic flourish. Serve the nuts as a tempting snack or a delightful appetizer.

Nutritional Benefits: Crunch and Flavor

Spiced roasted nuts offer a balance of crunch and warm flavors:

Mixed Nuts: Protein, healthy fats, vitamins, minerals, and antioxidants.

Spices: Aromatic warmth and potential health benefits.

Honey or Maple Syrup: Natural sweetness and depth of flavor.

Versatility: A Irresistible Treat

Enjoy your spiced roasted nuts as a satisfying and versatile snack. They're perfect for parties, movie nights, or whenever you're craving a flavorful crunch

.

Avocado and Black Bean Salsa

Ingredients: A Symphony of Freshness

Avocado: Choose ripe avocados, diced into bite-sized pieces, for their creamy texture.

Black Beans: Opt for cooked or canned black beans, drained and rinsed, for a hearty protein source.

Tomato: Diced tomato adds juicy sweetness and color.

Red Onion: Finely chopped red onion contributes a mild pungency.

Cilantro: Chopped cilantro lends a burst of freshness.

Lime: Zest and juice of lime for a zesty kick.

Jalapeno: Finely chopped jalapeno adds a hint of heat (adjust to your preference).

Garlic: Minced garlic for depth of flavor.

Olive Oil: Drizzle for a touch of richness.

Salt and Black Pepper: To enhance and balance flavors.

Preparation: Crafting Culinary Vibrancy

Combine Ingredients: In a mixing bowl, combine the diced avocado, black beans, diced tomato, finely chopped red onion, chopped cilantro, minced garlic, and finely chopped jalapeno.

Zest and Juice: Zest the lime over the bowl to infuse the salsa with citrus aroma. Squeeze the lime juice over the ingredients for a zesty brightness.

Drizzle and Season: Drizzle a bit of olive oil over the salsa for a hint of richness. Season with salt and black pepper to taste.

Gently Toss: Gently toss all the ingredients together to ensure they are evenly combined without smashing the avocado.

Chill: Cover the bowl and refrigerate the avocado and black bean salsa for about 30 minutes to allow the flavors to meld and develop.

Serve and Enjoy: Transfer the chilled salsa to a serving bowl. Serve with tortilla chips, as a topping for grilled proteins, or as a side dish for a fresh and vibrant meal.

Nutritional Benefits: Creaminess and Freshness

Avocado and black bean salsa offers a blend of creaminess and vibrancy:

Avocado: Healthy fats, vitamins, and creamy texture.

Black Beans: Protein, fiber, and essential nutrients.

Tomato and Lime: Juiciness, vitamins, and zesty brightness.

Versatility: A Flavorful Accompaniment

Enjoy your avocado and black bean salsa as a refreshing and versatile dish. It's perfect for gatherings, picnics, or as a light and wholesome snack.

Baked Sweet Potato Fries

Ingredients: A Fusion of Flavors

Sweet Potatoes: Choose fresh sweet potatoes, peeled and cut into uniform fry-like shapes, for their natural sweetness and vibrant color.

Olive Oil: Drizzle for roasting and a hint of richness.

Cornstarch: A light coating of cornstarch helps achieve crispy perfection.

Spices: Opt for a mix of smoked paprika, garlic powder, onion powder, and a pinch of cayenne for a burst of flavor.

Salt and Black Pepper: To enhance and balance flavors.

Fresh Herbs: Chopped fresh parsley or rosemary for an aromatic flourish.

Preparation: Crafting Culinary Crunch

Preheat Oven: Preheat your oven to 425°F (220°C) and line a baking sheet with parchment paper.

Toss with Cornstarch: In a bowl, toss the sweet potato fries with a light coating of cornstarch. This will help them become crispy when baked.

Drizzle with Olive Oil: Drizzle olive oil over the sweet potato fries and toss to coat them evenly. This will help the spices adhere and create a golden crispness.

Season with Spices: Sprinkle the smoked paprika, garlic powder, onion powder, cayenne (if using), salt, and black pepper over the fries. Toss again to ensure even distribution of the spices.

Arrange and Bake: Arrange the seasoned sweet potato fries in a single layer on the prepared baking sheet, ensuring they are not overcrowded. This will help them roast evenly and become crispy.

Roast to Perfection: Roast the sweet potato fries in the preheated oven for about 20-25 minutes, flipping them halfway through. Keep an eye on them to ensure they don't over-brown.

Garnish and Serve: Once the fries are golden and crispy, remove them from the oven. Garnish with chopped fresh herbs like parsley or rosemary. Serve the baked sweet potato fries hot.

Nutritional Benefits: Crispiness and Wholesomeness

Baked sweet potato fries offer a balance of crunch and nutrition:

Sweet Potatoes: Vitamins A and C, fiber, and natural sweetness.

Olive Oil: Healthy fats and richness.

Spices: Flavor depth and potential health benefits.

Versatility: A Crowd-Pleasing Side

Enjoy your baked sweet potato fries as a satisfying and versatile side dish. Serve them alongside burgers, sandwiches, or as a wholesome snack.

CHAPTER 6: DECADENT DESSERTS

Berry Parfait with Greek Yogurt

Ingredients: A Symphony of Sweetness

Greek Yogurt: Choose thick and creamy Greek yogurt for its tangy richness and protein content.

Assorted Berries: Opt for a mix of fresh berries such as strawberries, blueberries, raspberries, or blackberries for a colorful medley.

Honey or Maple Syrup: For a touch of natural sweetness.

Granola: Choose your favorite granola for a satisfying crunch.

Nuts or Seeds: Optional chopped nuts or seeds such as almonds, walnuts, or chia seeds for added texture.

Fresh Mint: Chopped mint leaves for an aromatic flourish.

Preparation: Crafting Culinary Elegance

Prepare Berries: Wash and gently dry the assorted berries. If using strawberries, hull and slice them.

Sweeten Yogurt: In a bowl, mix a drizzle of honey or maple syrup into the Greek yogurt to lightly sweeten it. Adjust the sweetness to your preference.

Assemble Layers: In serving glasses or bowls, start by layering a spoonful of the sweetened Greek yogurt at the bottom. Add a layer of mixed berries on top.

Add Crunch: Sprinkle a layer of granola over the berries for a satisfying crunch.

Repeat Layers: Continue layering with another spoonful of yogurt, more berries, and another layer of granola.

Garnish and Serve: Finish with a final layer of Greek yogurt. Garnish with chopped nuts or seeds and fresh mint leaves for an elegant touch.

Serve and Enjoy: Serve the berry parfait with Greek yogurt immediately, or refrigerate for a short while to let the flavors meld. Enjoy this delightful dessert with a spoonful of each layer in every bite.

Nutritional Benefits: Creaminess and Vibrancy

Berry parfait with Greek yogurt offers a blend of creaminess and natural sweetness:

Greek Yogurt: Protein, probiotics, and tangy richness.

Assorted Berries: Vitamins, antioxidants, and vibrant colors.

Granola and Nuts: Satisfying crunch and added nutrients.

Versatility: A Sweet Treat

Enjoy your berry parfait with Greek yogurt as a satisfying and versatile dessert. It's perfect for a quick sweet indulgence or as a delightful addition to brunch.

DarkChocolate-Dipped Strawberries

Ingredients: A Fusion of Indulgence

Fresh Strawberries: Choose ripe and plump strawberries, washed and thoroughly dried, for their natural sweetness.

Dark Chocolate: Opt for high-quality dark chocolate with at least 70% cocoa content for its deep richness.

Coconut Oil: A small amount of coconut oil helps the chocolate achieve a glossy finish and a smooth consistency.

Toppings: Optional toppings like chopped nuts, shredded coconut, or sprinkles for added texture and flair.

Preparation: Crafting Culinary Elegance

Melt Chocolate: In a heatproof bowl, melt the dark chocolate along with a small amount of coconut oil. You can use a microwave in short intervals or a double boiler on the stove. Stir until smooth and well combined.

Dip Strawberries: Hold a strawberry by the stem and dip it into the melted chocolate, coating about two-thirds of the berry. Allow any excess chocolate to drip off.

Add Toppings: If using toppings, immediately sprinkle them over the chocolate-coated part of the strawberry before the chocolate sets. This adds texture and visual appeal.

Set and Cool: Place the dipped strawberries on a parchment-lined tray or plate. Allow them to cool and set at room temperature. You can speed up the process by placing them in the refrigerator for a short while.

Serve and Enjoy: Once the chocolate has fully set, arrange the dark chocolate-dipped strawberries on a serving platter. Present them elegantly and serve as a delightful dessert or a luxurious treat.

Nutritional Benefits: Sweetness and Richness

Dark chocolate-dipped strawberries offer a blend of sweetness and richness:

Strawberries: Natural sweetness, vitamins, and antioxidants.

Dark Chocolate: Antioxidants, flavonoids, and indulgent richness.

Versatility: A Luxurious Delight

Enjoy your dark chocolate-dipped strawberries as a special dessert for celebrations, romantic occasions, or simply as a decadent treat to savor.

Cinnamon-Spiced Apple Crisp

Ingredients: A Symphony of Spice

Apples: Choose firm and tart apples such as Granny Smith, peeled, cored, and sliced, for their texture and flavor.

Cinnamon: Ground cinnamon adds warmth and aroma.

Brown Sugar: For a subtle caramel sweetness that complements the apples.

Lemon: Zest and juice of lemon for a bright contrast.

Flour: All-purpose flour for the crisp topping.

Oats: Rolled oats for added texture and heartiness.

Butter: Cold butter, diced, for a crisp and buttery topping.

Nuts: Optional chopped nuts such as walnuts or pecans for extra crunch.

Salt: To enhance and balance flavors.

Preparation: Crafting Culinary Comfort

Preheat Oven: Preheat your oven to 350°F (175°C).

Prepare Apples: In a bowl, toss the sliced apples with ground cinnamon, brown sugar, lemon zest, and a squeeze of lemon juice. Mix well to coat the apples with the fragrant spices.

Layer Apples: Transfer the spiced apples to a baking dish, spreading them evenly.

Prepare Crisp Topping: In a separate bowl, combine all-purpose flour, rolled oats, diced cold butter, chopped nuts (if using), and a pinch of salt. Use your fingertips to work the mixture until it resembles coarse crumbs.

Crisp Assembly: Sprinkle the crisp topping over the spiced apples, covering them evenly.

Bake: Place the baking dish in the preheated oven and bake for about 35-40 minutes, or until the topping is golden brown and the apples are tender.

Serve and Enjoy: Remove the cinnamon-spiced apple crisp from the oven and let it cool slightly. Serve the warm dessert with a scoop of vanilla ice cream or a dollop of whipped cream for a delightful treat.

Nutritional Benefits: Comfort and Flavor

Cinnamon-spiced apple crisp offers a balance of comfort and flavor:

Apples: Vitamins, fiber, and natural sweetness.

Cinnamon: Warmth, aroma, and potential health benefits.

Oats and Nuts: Texture, heartiness, and added nutrients.

Versatility: A Cozy Treat

Enjoy your cinnamon-spiced apple crisp as a heartwarming dessert for chilly evenings, family gatherings, or any time you crave a dose of comfort.

Chia Seed Pudding with Fresh Berries

Ingredients: A Symphony of Nutrients

Chia Seeds: Choose high-quality chia seeds for their gelatinous texture and nutritional benefits.

Milk: Opt for your choice of milk, such as almond milk, coconut milk, or dairy milk, for a creamy base.

Sweetener: Agave syrup, maple syrup, or honey for a touch of sweetness (adjust to taste).

Vanilla Extract: A dash of vanilla extract for aromatic depth.

Fresh Berries: Select an assortment of fresh berries like strawberries, blueberries, raspberries, or blackberries for vibrant colors and natural sweetness.

Nuts or Seeds: Optional chopped nuts or seeds such as almonds, walnuts, or pumpkin seeds for added texture and nutrients.

Preparation: Crafting Culinary Nourishment

Mix Chia Seeds and Liquid: In a bowl or jar, mix the chia seeds with the milk of your choice. Stir well to combine and prevent clumping. Allow the mixture to sit for a few minutes and then stir again to distribute the chia seeds evenly.

Sweeten and Flavor: Add a drizzle of sweetener (agave syrup, maple syrup, or honey) and a dash of vanilla extract to the chia seed and milk mixture. Stir to incorporate the flavors.

Chill and Set: Cover the bowl or jar and refrigerate the chia seed pudding for at least 2-3 hours, or preferably overnight. The chia seeds will absorb the liquid and create a pudding-like consistency.

Layer with Fresh Berries: Once the chia seed pudding has set, layer it in serving glasses or bowls with fresh berries. You can alternate between layers of pudding and layers of berries for a visually appealing presentation.

Garnish with Nuts or Seeds: If using nuts or seeds, sprinkle them over the top of the chia seed pudding and berries for added texture and a nutrient boost.

Serve and Enjoy: Serve the chia seed pudding with fresh berries as a nourishing dessert or a wholesome breakfast. Enjoy the balance of creamy chia pudding with the vibrant sweetness of the berries.

Nutritional Benefits: Wholesomeness and Flavor

Chia seed pudding with fresh berries offers a blend of wholesomeness and natural goodness:

Chia Seeds: Fiber, omega-3 fatty acids, and plant-based protein.

Milk: Calcium, vitamins, and creamy texture.

Berries: Vitamins, antioxidants, and vibrant colors.

Nuts or Seeds: Added nutrients, texture, and crunch.

Versatility: A Nutrient-Rich Treat

Enjoy your chia seed pudding with fresh berries as a versatile dessert, breakfast, or snack. It's a perfect way to start the day on a nutritious note or satisfy your sweet cravings guilt-free.

Portion Control and Carb Awareness

In the journey of managing diabetes, the concepts of portion control and carb awareness stand as pillars of empowerment. These principles offer a clear roadmap to maintain blood sugar levels and promote overall health. By understanding the impact of portion sizes and carbohydrate intake, individuals with diabetes can make informed choices that positively influence their well-being.

Portion Control: Right Size, Right Balance

Portion control is about recognizing that how much you eat matters just as much as what you eat. Maintaining balanced portions helps manage blood sugar levels, prevents overeating, and assists in weight management. It's essential to recognize that portion sizes may differ from what we're accustomed to, but the goal is to align with your body's needs.

Strategies for Portion Control:

Use Visual References: Familiarize yourself with visual cues to gauge portion sizes. For instance, a deck of cards represents a serving of meat, and a tennis ball equals a serving of fruit.

Choose Smaller Plates: Opt for smaller plates and bowls to create an illusion of fuller servings, helping prevent overeating.

Practice Mindful Eating: Slow down and savor each bite. This allows your body to signal when it's full.

Pre-Plate Meals: Portion out your meal before eating to prevent unconscious overeating from larger serving bowls.

Listen to Hunger Cues: Pay attention to your body's signals of hunger and fullness. Eat until you're satisfied, not overly full.

Carb Awareness: Balancing Blood Sugar

Carbohydrates significantly impact blood sugar levels, making carb awareness a fundamental aspect of diabetes management. While carbs are a vital energy source, managing their intake helps prevent spikes and crashes in blood sugar levels.

Strategies for Carb Awareness:

Identify Carb Sources: Learn to recognize foods rich in carbohydrates, including grains, fruits, starchy vegetables, and dairy products.

Count Carbs: Use carbohydrate counting to track your carb intake. This knowledge empowers you to adjust insulin doses or make dietary choices accordingly.

Prioritize Complex Carbs: Opt for complex carbohydrates like whole grains, legumes, and vegetables, which release energy gradually and have a milder impact on blood sugar levels.

Pair Carbs with Protein and Fiber: Combining carbs with protein and fiber slows down their digestion, helping maintain steady blood sugar levels.

Monitor Blood Sugar: Regular blood sugar monitoring gives you insights into how different foods affect your levels, allowing you to make informed choices.

The Benefits of Combining Portion Control and Carb Awareness:

Blood Sugar Stability: These strategies work in harmony to prevent rapid spikes and crashes in blood sugar levels, promoting overall stability.

Weight Management: Portion control prevents excess calorie consumption, supporting weight management—a crucial factor in diabetes control.

Empowerment: Both concepts empower individuals to take an active role in their health, fostering a sense of control and confidence.

Flexibility: Armed with portion control and carb awareness, you can still enjoy a variety of foods while managing your diabetes effectively.

Long-Term Health: Consistent application of these principles not only helps manage immediate blood sugar levels but also contributes to better long-term health outcomes.

In conclusion, the combination of portion control and carb awareness forms a dynamic duo for diabetes management. By embracing these principles, individuals with diabetes gain the tools to make mindful and well-informed choices that support blood sugar control, weight management, and overall well-being. With knowledge as your ally, you're empowered to navigate the world of nutrition and diabetes with confidence and success.

The Plate Method for Balanced Meals

The Plate Method is a practical and effective approach to creating balanced meals that promote optimal health and support various dietary goals, including diabetes management. This visual tool simplifies meal planning by using the proportions of a plate to guide your food choices, ensuring a well-rounded intake of nutrients while keeping portion sizes in check. Here's how the Plate Method works and why it's a valuable strategy for crafting balanced meals.

The Components of the Plate Method:

Half the Plate: Non-Starchy Vegetables: Fill half of your plate with a colorful assortment of non-starchy vegetables like leafy greens, broccoli, peppers, zucchini, and tomatoes. These veggies are low in carbohydrates and calories, yet rich in vitamins, minerals, and fiber.

One-Quarter of the Plate: Lean Protein: Dedicate one-quarter of your plate to lean protein sources such as poultry, fish, tofu, legumes, or eggs. Protein helps keep you full, supports muscle health, and has a minimal impact on blood sugar levels.

One-Quarter of the Plate: Whole Grains or Starchy Vegetables: Reserve the remaining quarter of your plate for whole grains like brown rice, quinoa, or whole wheat pasta, or starchy vegetables like sweet potatoes or corn. These provide energy through complex carbohydrates while offering essential nutrients and fiber.

Add a Side of Healthy Fat: Include a small serving of healthy fats like olive oil, nuts, or avocado. These fats contribute to satiety, aid nutrient absorption, and provide essential fatty acids.

Advantages of the Plate Method:

Simplicity: The Plate Method offers a simple and memorable visual guide for meal planning. Its straightforward approach makes it easy to apply to various meals and situations.

Balanced Nutrient Intake: By allocating space on your plate for different food groups, you naturally create a well-balanced meal with a variety of nutrients—carbohydrates, proteins, fats, vitamins, and minerals.

Portion Control: The Plate Method inherently emphasizes portion control. By following the proportions suggested, you're less likely to overeat, which is crucial for weight management and blood sugar control.

Flexibility: The Plate Method is adaptable to various dietary preferences and restrictions. It accommodates vegetarian, vegan, and gluten-free diets, making it a versatile tool for different individuals.

Mindful Choices: This method encourages mindfulness as you consider the composition of your plate. It prompts you to make conscious decisions about the foods you consume.

Applying the Plate Method for Balanced Meals:

Breakfast: Fill half your plate with berries, yogurt, and a small whole-grain muffin or toast with almond butter.

Lunch: Include a generous salad with mixed greens, grilled chicken (or tofu), quinoa, and a drizzle of olive oil vinaigrette.

Dinner: Enjoy a portion of baked salmon with steamed broccoli, roasted sweet potatoes, and a side of mixed nuts.

Snack: Create a mini-plate with carrot sticks, hummus, and a handful of whole-grain crackers.

Incorporating the Plate Method into your routine simplifies the process of crafting balanced meals that support your health goals, whether you're aiming for diabetes management, weight loss, or overall well-being. By embracing this practical approach, you can make informed food choices and nourish your body with a diverse array of nutrients in every meal.

Grocery Shopping Tips for Diabetes-Friendly Foods

Navigating the aisles of the grocery store can be a rewarding journey towards better health, especially when managing diabetes. Making thoughtful choices and selecting diabetes-friendly foods can positively impact blood sugar levels and overall well-being. Here are practical grocery shopping tips to help you fill your cart with nutritious and balanced options.

1. Plan Ahead:

Create a shopping list before heading to the store. Having a plan can prevent impulse purchases and guide you towards healthier choices.

2. Choose Whole Foods:

Prioritize whole foods like fresh fruits, vegetables, lean proteins, whole grains, and legumes. These foods are naturally rich in nutrients and fiber.

3. Embrace Fresh Produce:

Load up on colorful, non-starchy vegetables like leafy greens, peppers, cucumbers, and zucchini. These low-carb options are packed with vitamins and fiber.

4. Opt for Lean Proteins:

Select lean protein sources such as skinless poultry, fish, lean cuts of meat, tofu, tempeh, and legumes. Protein helps stabilize blood sugar levels and keeps you feeling full.

5. Incorporate Healthy Fats:

Choose sources of healthy fats like avocados, nuts, seeds, and olive oil. These fats promote heart health and help control blood sugar spikes.

6. Focus on Fiber:

Look for high-fiber options like whole grains (brown rice, quinoa, whole wheat pasta), legumes, and oats.

Fiber aids digestion and slows the absorption of sugars.

7. Check Labels:

Pay attention to nutrition labels. Aim for foods with lower added sugars, sodium, and saturated fats. Look for products with higher fiber content.

8. Limit Processed Foods:

Minimize processed foods like sugary cereals, snacks, and sugary beverages. These can lead to rapid spikes in blood sugar levels.

9. Choose Low-Fat Dairy:

Opt for low-fat or fat-free dairy options like Greek yogurt, milk, and cheese to reduce saturated fat intake.

10. Watch Portion Sizes:

Be mindful of portion sizes. Smaller portions help control calorie intake and maintain steady blood sugar levels.

11. Prioritize Unprocessed Snacks:

Choose snacks like whole fruits, vegetables with hummus, nuts, or low-fat yogurt. These options provide sustained energy without spiking blood sugar.

12. Shop the Perimeter:

Spend more time in the outer aisles of the store, where fresh produce, lean proteins, dairy, and whole grains are usually located.

13. Be Mindful of Sugars:

Check ingredient lists for added sugars. Look for different names like sucrose, high-fructose corn syrup, and agave nectar.

14. Consider Frozen Options:

Frozen fruits and vegetables can be just as nutritious as fresh ones and can be a convenient option to have on hand.

15. Stay Hydrated:

Include sugar-free beverages like water, herbal tea, or sparkling water in your shopping list to stay hydrated without extra sugars.

16. Read Labels on Sauces and Condiments:

Check the nutrition labels on sauces and condiments. Opt for lower-sugar or reduced-sodium options.

17. Shop When You're Not Hungry:

Shopping on an empty stomach can lead to impulse purchases of less healthy foods.

By applying these grocery shopping tips, you'll not only be making diabetes-friendly choices but also fostering a healthier lifestyle overall. Remember, a well-stocked pantry and fridge with nutritious options can make it easier to create balanced and delicious meals that support your diabetes management goals.

Weekly Meal Planning Guide

Meal planning is a powerful tool for maintaining a balanced and nutritious diet, especially when managing diabetes. By thoughtfully planning your meals for the week ahead, you can make informed choices, reduce stress, save time, and support your health goals. Here's a comprehensive weekly meal planning guide to help you create nourishing and diabetes-friendly meals.

1. Set Your Goals:

Define your health goals, whether it's blood sugar management, weight loss, or overall well-being. Tailor your meals to align with these objectives.

2. Inventory and Planning:

Take inventory of your pantry, fridge, and freezer. Note what ingredients you have and what needs replenishing.

3. Create a Meal Planning Template:

Use a template that outlines breakfast, lunch, dinner, and snacks for each day of the week. You can use a digital tool, a notebook, or a printable template.

4. Include Balanced Meals:

Aim to create balanced meals that incorporate protein, healthy fats, complex carbs, and fiber. Think about the Plate Method: non-starchy vegetables, lean protein, whole grains/starchy veggies, and a side of healthy fats.

5. Utilize Leftovers:

Plan meals that use ingredients in multiple dishes to reduce waste. Leftovers can become the base for the next day's lunch or dinner.

6. Mix Up Protein Sources:

Vary your protein sources throughout the week. Include lean meats, poultry, fish, eggs, tofu, tempeh, legumes, and low-fat dairy.

7. Incorporate Whole Grains:

Integrate whole grains like brown rice, quinoa, whole wheat pasta, and oats into your meals. They provide sustained energy and fiber.

8. Embrace Non-Starchy Vegetables:

Fill half your plate with colorful non-starchy vegetables like spinach, broccoli, peppers, and cauliflower.

9. Plan Snacks:

Include diabetes-friendly snacks like nuts, Greek yogurt, cut veggies with hummus, or a piece of fruit.

10. Portion Control:

Be mindful of portion sizes. Consider using measuring cups or your hand as a reference.

11. Prep Ahead:

Dedicate a day (like the weekend) for meal prep. Chop veggies, cook grains, and pre-portion snacks for the week.

12. Think Variety:

Include a variety of foods to ensure you're getting a range of nutrients. Experiment with different recipes and cuisines.

13. Keep Special Occasions in Mind:

If you have special occasions or social gatherings planned, adjust your meal plan to accommodate them.

14. Check the Calendar:

Consider your schedule. Plan simpler meals on busy days and more elaborate ones when you have more time.

15. Grocery Shopping:

Create a detailed shopping list based on your meal plan. Stick to your list to avoid impulse purchases.

16. Stay Hydrated:

Include water as a vital component of your plan. Stay hydrated throughout the day.

17. Stay Flexible:

Life can be unpredictable. It's okay to make adjustments to your meal plan if needed.

18. Evaluate and Adjust:

At the end of the week, assess how well your plan worked. Note what worked and what you'd like to change for the following week.

Sample Weekly Meal Plan:

Monday:

Breakfast: Greek yogurt with berries and a sprinkle of nuts.

Lunch: Grilled chicken salad with mixed greens, cucumbers, tomatoes, and a light vinaigrette.

Snack: Carrot sticks with hummus.

Dinner: Baked salmon with quinoa and steamed broccoli.

Tuesday:

Breakfast: Oatmeal topped with sliced banana and a drizzle of almond butter.

Lunch: Lentil and vegetable soup with whole grain crackers.

Snack: Apple slices with a small portion of cheese.

Dinner: Stir-fried tofu with mixed veggies and brown rice.

Wednesday:

Breakfast: Scrambled eggs with spinach and whole grain toast.

Lunch: Quinoa salad with mixed vegetables, chickpeas, and a light lemon vinaigrette.

Snack: Handful of mixed nuts.

Dinner: Grilled turkey burgers with sweet potato wedges and a side salad.

Thursday:

Breakfast: Whole grain waffles topped with Greek yogurt and fresh berries.

Lunch: Wrap filled with lean turkey slices, avocado, lettuce, and tomato.

Snack: Cottage cheese with pineapple chunks.

Dinner: Baked chicken with roasted Brussels sprouts and a side of quinoa.

Friday:

Breakfast: Smoothie with spinach, banana, unsweetened almond milk, and a scoop of protein powder.

Lunch: Whole grain pasta salad with cherry tomatoes, black olives, and feta cheese.

Snack: Rice cakes with almond butter.

Dinner: Fish tacos with whole wheat tortillas, coleslaw, and a side of black beans.

Saturday:

Breakfast: Veggie omelette with a side of whole grain toast.

Lunch: Hummus and vegetable wrap with a side of carrot sticks.

Snack: Greek yogurt with a drizzle of honey.

Dinner: Stir-fried shrimp with mixed vegetables and brown rice.

<u>Sunday:</u>

Breakfast: Overnight chia seed pudding with mixed berries.

Lunch: Spinach and mixed greens salad with grilled chicken, walnuts, and balsamic vinaigrette.

Snack: Sliced pear with a small piece of cheese.

Dinner: Roasted vegetable and quinoa bowl with a tahini dressing.

Remember, this sample meal plan is just a starting point. Customize it based on your dietary preferences, nutritional needs, and lifestyle. Feel free to swap out ingredients, adjust portion sizes, and experiment with new recipes. Consistency and balance are key when managing diabetes through your diet. Enjoy your journey to better health through mindful meal planning!

CHAPTER 8: LIFESTYLE TIPS FOR MANAGING DIABETES

Staying Active and Incorporating Exercise

Regular physical activity is a cornerstone of managing diabetes and promoting overall well-being. Exercise helps control blood sugar levels, boosts cardiovascular health, enhances insulin sensitivity, and contributes to weight management. Whether you're new to exercise or looking to revamp your routine, here's a comprehensive guide to staying active and incorporating exercise into your daily life.

1. Choose Activities You Enjoy:

Opt for activities you find enjoyable, whether it's walking, swimming, cycling, dancing, yoga, or playing a sport. When you enjoy what you're doing, you're more likely to stick with it.

2. Start Slowly:

If you're new to exercise, start slowly and gradually increase intensity and duration. Consult your healthcare provider before beginning a new exercise regimen, especially if you have any medical conditions.

3. Set Realistic Goals:

Set achievable goals that are specific, measurable, attainable, relevant, and time-bound (SMART). This could be walking for 30 minutes a day or trying a new exercise class twice a week.

4. Prioritize Consistency:

Consistency is key. Aim for regular exercise, even if it's just 15-30 minutes a day. Building a routine helps make exercise a habit.

5. Mix It Up:

Incorporate a variety of exercises to keep things interesting and target different muscle groups. This prevents boredom and plateaus.

6. Cardiovascular Exercise:

Engage in cardiovascular activities like brisk walking, jogging, cycling, or swimming. Aim for at least 150 minutes of moderate-intensity aerobic exercise per week.

7. Strength Training:

Include strength training exercises to build muscle and improve metabolism. Focus on major muscle groups with activities like weight lifting, resistance bands, or bodyweight exercises.

8. Flexibility and Balance:

Practice flexibility exercises like yoga or stretching to improve range of motion and balance. This can help prevent injuries and enhance overall well-being.

9. Monitor Blood Sugar Levels:

Check your blood sugar before and after exercise to understand how your body responds. Learn how exercise affects your levels and adjust your routine accordingly.

10. Stay Hydrated:

Drink water before, during, and after exercise to stay hydrated. Dehydration can affect blood sugar levels.

11. Warm Up and Cool Down:

Begin each exercise session with a warm-up to gradually increase heart rate and circulation. End with a cool-down to help your body recover.

12. Listen to Your Body:

Pay attention to how your body feels during and after exercise. If you feel dizzy, lightheaded, or experience discomfort, stop and rest.

13. Stay Mindful of Your Feet:

If you have diabetic neuropathy, wear appropriate footwear and choose low-impact activities to protect your feet.

14. Consider Timing:

Experiment with different times of day to see when you feel most energized and motivated to exercise.

15. Make it Social:

Engage in group activities, exercise classes, or workouts with friends. Social support can keep you motivated and accountable.

16. Track Your Progress:

Keep a journal or use fitness apps to track your workouts, set goals, and celebrate your achievements.

17. Adapt to Your Schedule:

If you have a busy day, break your exercise into shorter bouts. Even 10-minute bursts of activity can add up.

18. Celebrate Small Wins:

Celebrate your achievements, no matter how small. Every step towards a more active lifestyle is a positive move.

Remember, the journey to a more active lifestyle is personal. Listen to your body, respect your limits, and find joy in the process. Consistency and gradual progress are key to reaping the long-term benefits of exercise on your diabetes management and overall health.

Stress Management and Its Impact on Blood Sugar

Stress is a natural part of life, but when it becomes chronic or overwhelming, it can have significant implications for your health, especially if you're managing diabetes. Stress can affect blood sugar levels and complicate diabetes management. Understanding the connection between stress and blood sugar and adopting effective stress management techniques are essential for maintaining overall well-being.

The Stress-Blood Sugar Connection:

Stress triggers the release of hormones like cortisol and adrenaline, which can lead to an increase in blood sugar levels. This physiological response is often referred to as the "fight or flight" response, designed to provide energy for immediate action. However, when stress is persistent, these hormonal changes can disrupt blood sugar regulation in individuals with diabetes.

Impact of Stress on Diabetes Management:

Blood Sugar Spikes: Stress-induced blood sugar spikes can make diabetes management more challenging, as it may require adjustments to medication or insulin doses.

Decreased Insulin Sensitivity: Chronic stress can lead to decreased insulin sensitivity, making it harder for your body to use insulin effectively.

Emotional Eating: Stress can lead to emotional eating, causing individuals to choose less healthy food options and overeat, which can affect blood sugar control.

Lifestyle Changes: High stress levels can lead to neglecting healthy habits like exercise, balanced meals, and regular sleep—all of which play a crucial role in diabetes management.

Effective Stress Management Techniques:

Practice Mindfulness and Meditation:

Mindfulness and meditation techniques can help you stay present and manage stress. Deep breathing exercises, progressive muscle relaxation, and guided meditation can promote relaxation and reduce stress levels.

Engage in Physical Activity:

Regular exercise has been shown to reduce stress and improve mood. Choose activities you enjoy, whether it's walking, yoga, dancing, or swimming.

Prioritize Sleep:

Quality sleep is vital for managing stress. Establish a sleep routine, create a comfortable sleep environment, and aim for 7-9 hours of sleep each night.

Stay Connected:

Maintain strong social connections with friends and family. Talking about your feelings and concerns with loved ones can provide emotional support.

Limit Caffeine and Alcohol:

Excessive caffeine and alcohol consumption can worsen stress and affect sleep. Moderation is key.

Engage in Hobbies:

Pursue activities you're passionate about. Engaging in hobbies can provide a sense of accomplishment and relaxation.

Set Realistic Goals:

Avoid overloading yourself with tasks. Set achievable goals and break larger tasks into smaller, manageable steps.

Seek Professional Help:

If stress becomes overwhelming, consider speaking to a therapist or counselor. They can provide strategies to manage stress and improve emotional well-being.

The Importance of Self-Care:

Self-care is a crucial aspect of stress management. Allocate time for activities that nourish your mind, body, and soul. This could include reading, taking a relaxing bath, spending time in nature, or practicing a creative hobby.

In Conclusion: While stress is an inevitable part of life, managing it effectively can positively impact your diabetes management and overall health. By incorporating stress management techniques into your routine, you can better control your blood sugar levels, improve insulin sensitivity, and cultivate a sense of balance and well-being. Remember, taking care of your mental and emotional health is just as important as managing your physical health when it comes to diabetes management.

Sleep's Role in Diabetes Management

Quality sleep is a cornerstone of overall health and plays a significant role in diabetes management. Sleep impacts blood sugar control, insulin sensitivity, and various metabolic processes. Understanding the relationship between sleep and diabetes, as well as adopting healthy sleep habits, can contribute to more effective diabetes management and improved well-being.

The Sleep-Diabetes Connection:

Blood Sugar Regulation: Adequate sleep supports stable blood sugar levels. Sleep deprivation can lead to insulin resistance, making it harder for your cells to respond to insulin and regulate blood sugar effectively.

Hormone Regulation: Sleep affects the release of hormones that influence hunger and appetite, such as leptin and ghrelin. Poor sleep can lead to imbalances in these hormones, potentially causing overeating and weight gain.

Inflammation: Lack of sleep is associated with increased inflammation in the body, which can contribute to insulin resistance and other health issues.

Stress Management: Quality sleep helps manage stress levels. Chronic stress can impact blood sugar control and complicate diabetes management.

Tips for Improving Sleep Quality:

Establish a Consistent Sleep Schedule:

Go to bed and wake up at the same time every day, even on weekends. This helps regulate your body's internal clock.

Create a Relaxing Bedtime Routine:

Engage in calming activities before bed, such as reading, taking a warm bath, or practicing relaxation techniques.

Limit Screen Time Before Bed:

The blue light emitted by phones, tablets, and computers can interfere with your body's production of melatonin, a hormone that regulates sleep.

Create a Comfortable Sleep Environment:

Ensure your bedroom is dark, quiet, and at a comfortable temperature. Invest in a supportive mattress and pillows.

Limit Caffeine and Alcohol Intake:

Avoid caffeine and alcohol close to bedtime, as they can disrupt sleep patterns.

Stay Active During the Day:

Regular physical activity can improve sleep quality. However, avoid vigorous exercise close to bedtime.

Watch Your Diet:

Avoid heavy or spicy meals before bed, as they can cause discomfort and disrupt sleep.

Manage Stress:

Practice stress-reduction techniques, such as meditation, deep breathing, or gentle yoga, to promote relaxation.

Limit Naps:

If you nap during the day, keep it short (20-30 minutes) and avoid napping too close to bedtime.

Limit Fluid Intake Before Bed:

To prevent waking up in the middle of the night to use the restroom, limit your fluid intake in the evening.

The Benefits of Prioritizing Sleep:

Improved Blood Sugar Control: Quality sleep can lead to better blood sugar regulation and reduced insulin resistance.

Enhanced Insulin Sensitivity: Adequate sleep improves your body's ability to use insulin effectively.

Weight Management: Balanced sleep supports healthy metabolism and reduces the likelihood of overeating.

Mood and Mental Health: Quality sleep contributes to emotional well-being and cognitive function.

Overall Well-Being: Consistent, restful sleep enhances your overall quality of life.

<u>In Conclusion,</u> Quality sleep is a fundamental component of effective diabetes management. By prioritizing restful sleep and adopting healthy sleep habits, you can optimize blood sugar control, insulin sensitivity, and various aspects of your health. Consider your sleep routine as an integral part of your diabetes management plan, supporting your journey towards well-being and improved quality of life.

Building a Supportive Diabetes Care Team

Managing diabetes effectively requires a comprehensive approach that extends beyond individual efforts. A supportive diabetes care team can provide valuable guidance, expertise, and encouragement throughout your journey. By assembling a team of healthcare professionals, you can access a wealth of knowledge and resources to enhance your diabetes management and overall well-being. Here's how to build and utilize a strong diabetes care team:

Primary Care Physician (PCP) or Endocrinologist:

Your PCP or endocrinologist is a central figure in your care team. They oversee your diabetes management plan, prescribe medications, and coordinate your overall health.

Certified Diabetes Educator (CDE):

A CDE provides personalized education and guidance on managing diabetes. They can help you understand blood sugar monitoring, medication management, meal planning, and more.

Registered Dietitian (RD) or Nutritionist:

An RD can help you create a diabetes-friendly meal plan, manage portion sizes, and make healthier food choices to support blood sugar control and overall health.

Pharmacist:

Your pharmacist can provide insights on medications, potential interactions, and how different drugs may affect your diabetes management.

Exercise Specialist or Physical Therapist:

These professionals can design safe and effective exercise routines tailored to your needs and help you maintain an active lifestyle.

Mental Health Professional:

Managing diabetes involves emotional and psychological well-being. A therapist or counselor can provide strategies to cope with stress, anxiety, and other emotional challenges.

Ophthalmologist and Podiatrist:

Regular eye exams with an ophthalmologist help monitor diabetic retinopathy, while a podiatrist can help prevent and manage foot complications.

Dentist:

Diabetes can impact oral health. Regular dental check-ups are essential to prevent gum disease and other dental issues.

Social Support:

Friends, family, support groups, and online communities can provide emotional support, understanding, and shared experiences.

Health Apps and Technology:

Utilize diabetes management apps, glucose monitors, and wearable devices to track your progress and stay connected with your care team.

Steps to Building Your Diabetes Care Team:

1. Identify Your Needs:

Consider the areas of diabetes management where you need the most assistance or guidance. This will help you determine the types of professionals to include in your care team.

2. Ask for Recommendations:

Your primary care physician, healthcare network, or local diabetes organizations can recommend qualified professionals.

3. Check Credentials:

Verify the qualifications, certifications, and experience of each team member to ensure they are well-equipped to provide diabetes care.

4. Communication and Collaboration:

Encourage your care team members to communicate and collaborate with each other. This ensures everyone is on the same page and working towards your well-being.

5. Regular Check-Ins:

Schedule regular appointments with each team member to monitor progress, address concerns, and adjust your diabetes management plan as needed.

6. Be Open and Honest:

Share your experiences, challenges, and goals openly with your care team. This information helps them tailor their guidance to your unique needs.

7. Stay Educated:

Continue to educate yourself about diabetes management through reputable sources, so you can actively participate in decisions regarding your care.

8. Advocate for Yourself:

You are the central figure in your diabetes management. Don't hesitate to ask questions, seek clarification, and express your preferences to your care team.

Building a supportive diabetes care team is a crucial step towards effective diabetes management and overall well-being. These professionals provide a diverse range of expertise and perspectives to help you navigate the challenges of diabetes and make informed decisions. By working together with your care team, you can achieve better blood sugar control, prevent complications, and lead a healthier and more fulfilling life.

CONCLUSION

In the journey of managing diabetes, you've gained a deeper understanding of the intricacies involved in achieving optimal health and well-being. From the importance of balanced nutrition to the impact of exercise, stress, sleep, and the value of a supportive care team, you've explored a holistic approach that encompasses every facet of your life. By integrating these insights into your lifestyle, you're empowered to take charge of your health and make informed choices that positively influence your diabetes management.

Remember that managing diabetes is not just about numbers and medications; it's about fostering a mindful relationship with your body, nourishing it with nutritious foods, staying active to improve your physical vitality, and nurturing your emotional well-being. Each decision you make is a step towards a healthier future, and every small achievement contributes to the bigger picture of your wellness journey.

As you navigate the path ahead, keep in mind that setbacks may occur, but they don't define your progress. Approach challenges with resilience, seek support from your care team and loved ones, and continue to educate yourself. Your commitment to your health is a testament to your determination and strength.

In the tapestry of diabetes management, you are the weaver, crafting a life of balance, vitality, and fulfillment. Embrace the lessons learned, the habits formed, and the connections made on this journey. With knowledge, dedication, and the right resources, you have the power to live a vibrant life, filled with the richness of well-being and the joy of flavor-filled choices. Your journey towards flavorful living is a testament to your enduring commitment to your health, and you're on a path that leads to a brighter, healthier, and more fulfilling future.

Your Flavorful Diabetes Journey Ahead

As you stand at the threshold of your diabetes journey, armed with insights and a holistic approach, a world of flavorful possibilities awaits you. This journey is not just about managing diabetes; it's about reclaiming your health, embracing a vibrant lifestyle, and savoring every moment. You're equipped with the tools to make informed choices, and you have the strength to overcome any challenges that come your way.

Picture your path ahead as a canvas waiting to be painted with your unique experiences. With each wholesome meal, energizing exercise, moment of mindfulness, and connection forged with your care team, you're adding vibrant hues to this canvas. Your journey is a work of art that reflects your dedication, resilience, and the beauty of a life well-lived.

Amidst the twists and turns, remember that you're not alone. Your supportive care team, loved ones, and the knowledge you've gained are your companions on this adventure. Embrace the journey with an open heart and a curious mind. Explore new recipes that tantalize your taste buds while keeping your health in mind. Embrace physical activities that invigorate your body and elevate your spirits. Cultivate inner peace through mindfulness and stress management techniques. Cherish the restful nights that fuel your vitality.

Every step you take is a testament to your commitment to well-being. Your journey is as unique as your fingerprint, and it's an ongoing exploration of self-care, growth, and empowerment.

It's a testament to your strength, resilience, and the power you hold to shape your destiny.

So, stride forward with confidence and purpose. Embrace the flavors of life with zest and enthusiasm. Let your diabetes journey be a source of inspiration, not only for you but for others who witness your dedication. Your journey holds the promise of a healthier, more vibrant, and flavorful life—one that radiates well-being in every aspect.

With your heart set on wellness and your mind attuned to balance, you're ready to embark on this flavorful diabetes journey with courage, grace, and determination. As you move forward, may your path be paved with positive choices, enriching experiences, and a life that truly savors the art of living well.

Testimonials from Those Who Found Success

Testimonials from Those Who Found Success: Inspiring Stories of Triumph and Transformation

Real stories from real individuals who have walked the path of managing diabetes offer invaluable insights and inspiration. These testimonials serve as reminders that with dedication, knowledge, and a holistic approach, living well with diabetes is not only achievable but also deeply rewarding. Here are a few testimonials from individuals who found success on their diabetes journey:

Sarah's Story: Rediscovering Joy in Every Bite

"Managing diabetes felt like a daunting task at first, but I realized that it was a journey of self-discovery and empowerment. By embracing a balanced diet that includes vibrant vegetables, lean proteins, and wholesome grains, I found that I could enjoy delicious meals that support my health. From hearty breakfasts to satisfying dinners, each day became an opportunity to nourish my body and savor every bite. With the guidance of my care team, I not only improved my blood sugar control but also reignited my love for food and life."

John's Journey: From Sedentary to Strong

"Exercise wasn't always a part of my routine, but I soon realized its incredible impact on my diabetes management. Through gradual progress and consistent effort, I incorporated daily walks, strength training, and yoga into my life. Not only did my blood sugar levels stabilize, but I also felt a newfound vitality. I learned that exercise isn't a chore—it's an opportunity to nurture my body, boost my mood, and embrace a healthier lifestyle. My journey from being sedentary to becoming strong has been transformative, and I now look forward to each active moment."

Emily's Experience: Finding Balance in Mind and Body

"Stress used to take a toll on my well-being and blood sugar control. However, through mindfulness practices and stress management techniques, I've discovered the power of emotional balance. By engaging in meditation, deep breathing, and positive self-talk, I've not only reduced my stress levels but also gained a deeper connection with myself. It's incredible how nurturing my mental health positively impacts my physical health. I'm on a journey of holistic well-being, and it's a rewarding path filled with self-care and self-discovery."

Steve's Success: Thriving with Support

"Building a diabetes care team was a game-changer for me. With the guidance of healthcare professionals, a dietitian, and a supportive community, I've learned to navigate diabetes with confidence. From understanding portion control to managing stress and staying active, each member of my team has contributed to my success. The camaraderie, knowledge, and encouragement I receive inspire me to embrace life fully and prioritize my health."

These testimonials are a testament to the transformative power of embracing a holistic approach to diabetes management. Each story reflects the unique challenges, triumphs, and lessons that come with the journey. Through their experiences, these individuals remind us that diabetes management is not a limitation but an opportunity for growth, empowerment, and flavorful living. Their journeys offer insights, inspiration, and a guiding light for anyone navigating the path of diabetes with determination and grace.

Resources and Further Reading

Empowering yourself with knowledge is a cornerstone of effective diabetes management. As you continue your journey towards optimal health and well-being, the following resources and reading materials can provide you with valuable insights, guidance, and support:

1. American Diabetes Association (ADA):

Website: diabetes.org

ADA offers a wealth of information on diabetes management, healthy eating, physical activity, and more.

2. Mayo Clinic:

Website:mayoclinic.org/diseases-conditions/diabetes

Mayo Clinic provides comprehensive articles and resources on diabetes, its causes, symptoms, and management.

3. Centers for Disease Control and Prevention (CDC):

Website: cdc.gov/diabetes

CDC offers educational materials, statistics, and tips for preventing and managing diabetes.

4. WebMD Diabetes Center:

Website: webmd.com/diabetes

WebMD offers articles, videos, and interactive tools to help you understand and manage diabetes.

5. Diabetes Forecast Magazine:

Website: diabetesforecast.org

This publication by ADA provides expert advice, recipes, success stories, and the latest advancements in diabetes care.

6. "The Diabetes Code" by Dr. Jason Fung:

A book that delves into the science of diabetes, insulin resistance, and practical strategies for managing blood sugar.

7. "Think Like a Pancreas" by Gary Scheiner:

This book offers insights into diabetes management, including meal planning, insulin strategies, and troubleshooting.

8. "Diabetes for Dummies" by Alan L. Rubin:

A comprehensive guide that covers diabetes basics, management, and lifestyle adjustments.

9. Diabetes Support Groups and Online Communities:

Joining local support groups or online communities can provide you with a platform to connect with others managing diabetes, share experiences, and learn from one another.

10. Healthcare Professionals:

Your primary care physician, endocrinologist, certified diabetes educator, registered dietitian, and other healthcare professionals are valuable sources of personalized guidance and information.

11. Diabetes Management Apps:

Explore diabetes management apps that can help you track blood sugar levels, monitor food intake, and set reminders for medications and appointments.

12. Online Cooking Classes and Recipe Blogs:

Discover cooking classes and recipe blogs that focus on diabetes-friendly meals, allowing you to explore new flavors while prioritizing your health.

Remember that knowledge is a continuous journey. Stay curious, stay informed, and stay engaged in your diabetes management. As you explore these resources, you'll equip yourself with the tools and insights needed to lead a flavorful, balanced, and vibrant life while effectively managing diabetes. Your commitment to learning and empowerment is a testament to your dedication to well-being.

9 7 9 8 8 5 8 0 7 8 1 2 8